MY BODY AND ME

My Strong Muscles

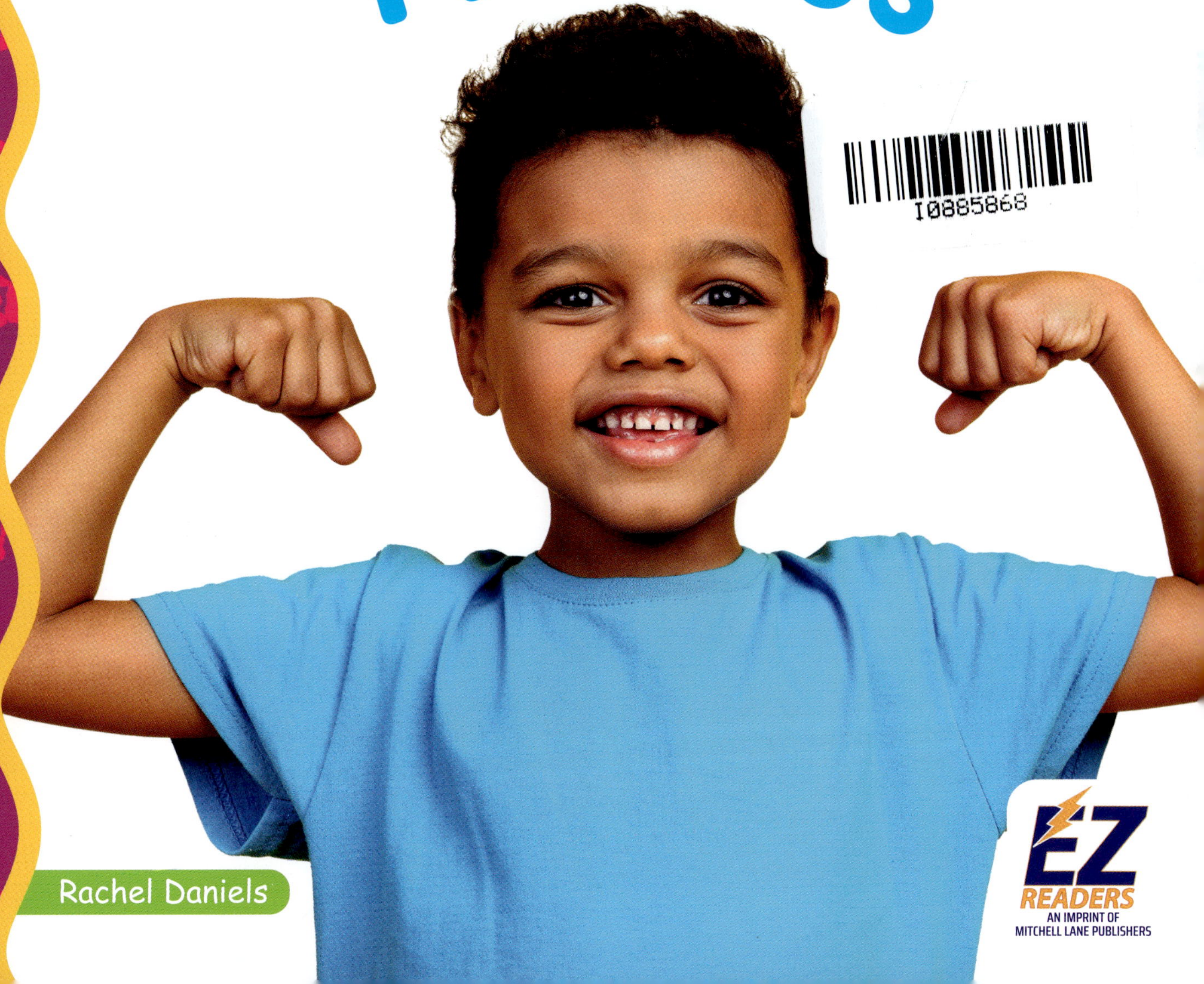

Rachel Daniels

EZ READERS
AN IMPRINT OF
MITCHELL LANE PUBLISHERS

CREATING YOUNG NONFICTION READERS

EZ Readers offer nonfiction for beginning readers in PreK through first grade, using simple language, clear illustrations, and engaging facts to build vocabulary and confidence.

TIPS FOR READING NONFICTION WITH BEGINNING READERS

Talk about Nonfiction

Begin by explaining that nonfiction books give us information that is true. The book will be organized around a specific topic or idea, and we may learn new facts through reading.

Look at the Parts

Most nonfiction books have helpful features. Our *EZ Readers* include color photographs and graphic aids, a table of contents, a glossary, and an index. Share the purpose of these features with your reader.

Color Photos and Graphic Aids

A lot of information can be found by "reading" photos, charts, maps, and other graphic aids found within nonfiction texts. Help your reader learn more about the different ways information can be displayed.

Table of Contents

Located at the front of the book, this list shows the big ideas within the text and the page numbers where they can be found.

Glossary

Located at the back of the book, the glossary defines key words and phrases that are related to the topic. These words and phrases can be found in the text in colored type.

Index

Located at the back of the book, an index is an alphabetical list of topics and the page numbers where they can be found.

With a little help and guidance about reading nonfiction, you can feel good about introducing a young reader to the world of *EZ Readers* nonfiction books.

EZ Readers is an imprint of:

Mitchell Lane
PUBLISHERS

2001 SW 31st Avenue
Hallandale, FL 33009
mitchelllanepub.com

First Edition, 2026.

Author: Rachel Daniels
Editor: Morgan Brody

ISBN 979-8-89260-829-9 (library binding)
ISBN 979-8-90145-035-2 (paperback)
ISBN 979-8-89260-830-5 (ebook)

LC record available at https://lccn.loc.gov/2025950868

Photo credits: Shutterstock, Alex Konon, cover, 1, 2, 3, 6, 11, 15, 16, 19, 20; Shutterstock, yusuf_demirci, cover, 1; iStock, Deagreez, cover, 1, 22; Designed by Freepik, 3, 7, 8, 11, 15; Shutterstock, alexkatkov, 4–5, 22; iStock, FatCamera, 7; iStock, FamVeld, 8, 22; Shutterstock, PeopleImages, 10, 22; Shutterstock, Sergey Novikov, 12–13; iStock, FabrikaCr, 14, 22; iStock, MangoStar_Studio, 17, 22; iStock, FatCamera, 18, 22; Shutterstock, Africa Studio, 21; Shutterstock, PeopleImages, 22

Table of Contents

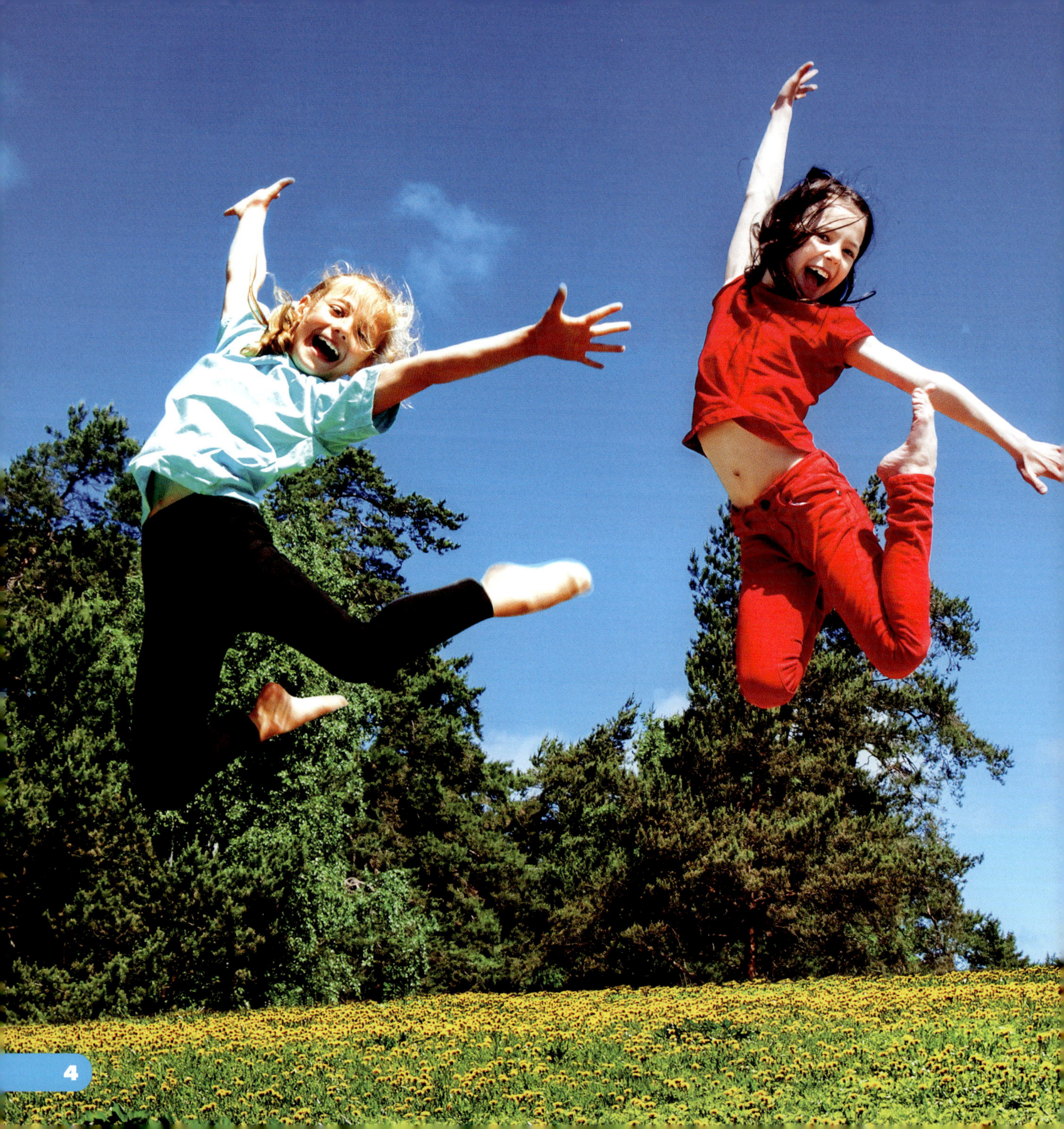

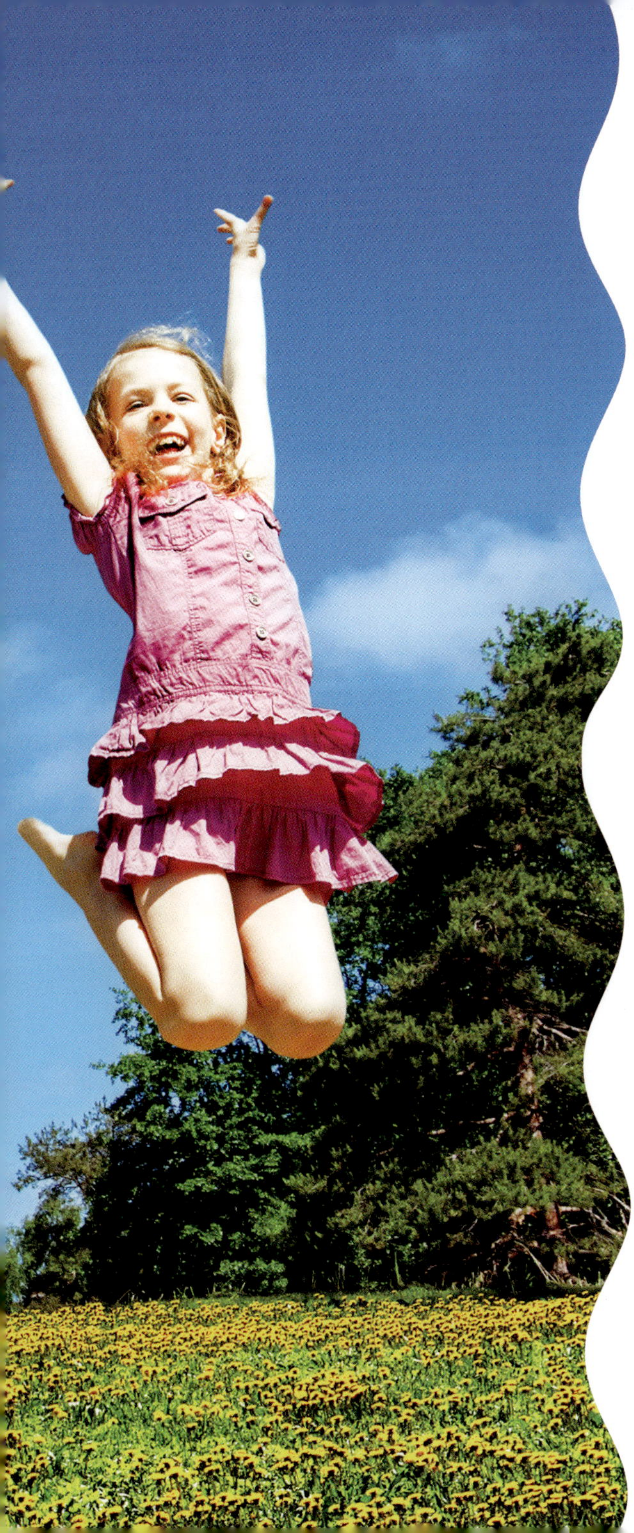

I move my arms.

I move my legs.

I run. I jump. I dance.

Muscles help me move!

Muscles Everywhere

I have muscles all over.

I have muscles in my arms.

I have muscles in my legs.

I have muscles in my face.

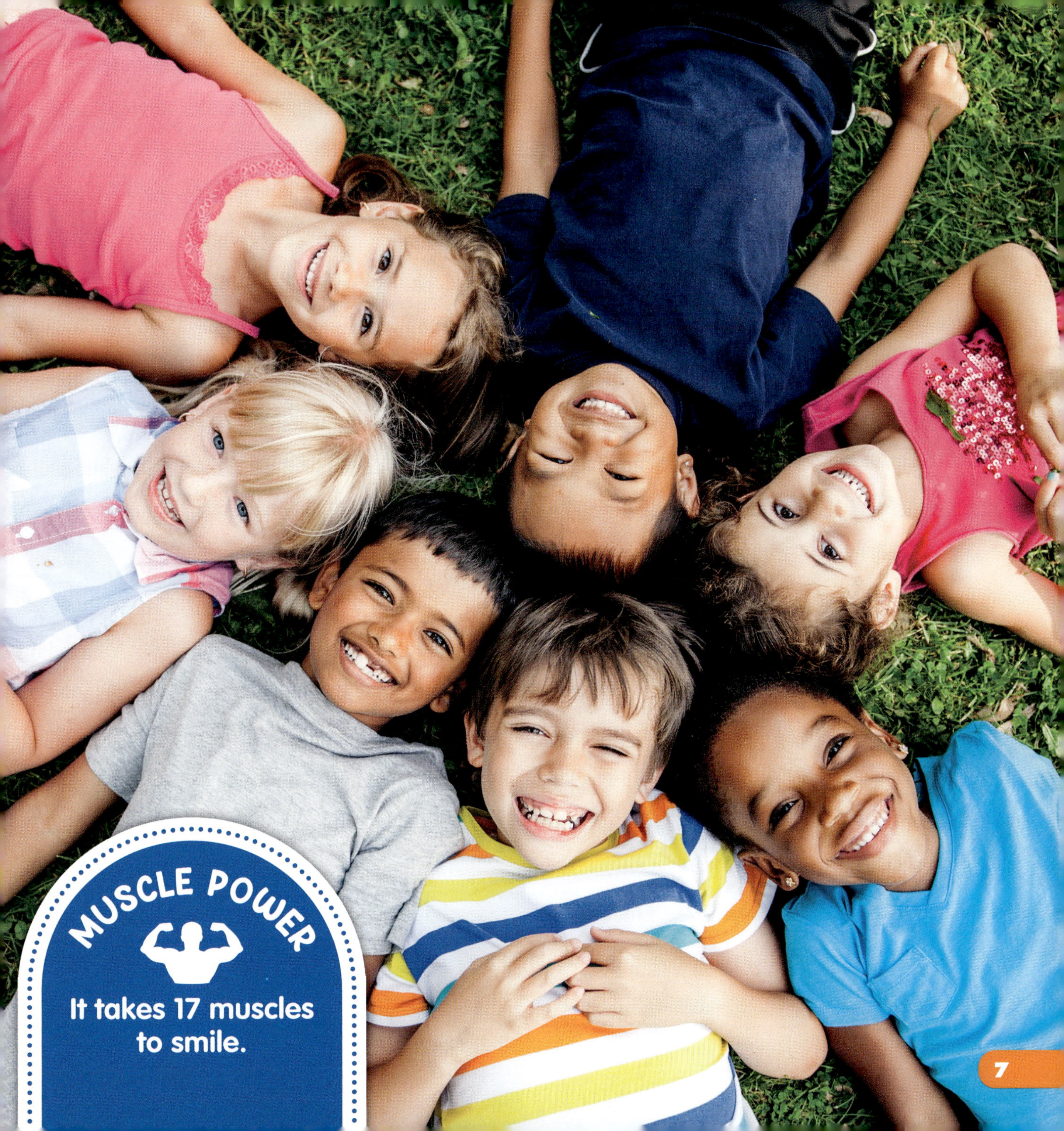

MUSCLE POWER

It takes 17 muscles to smile.

MUSCLE POWER

The biggest muscle is my **thigh** muscle.

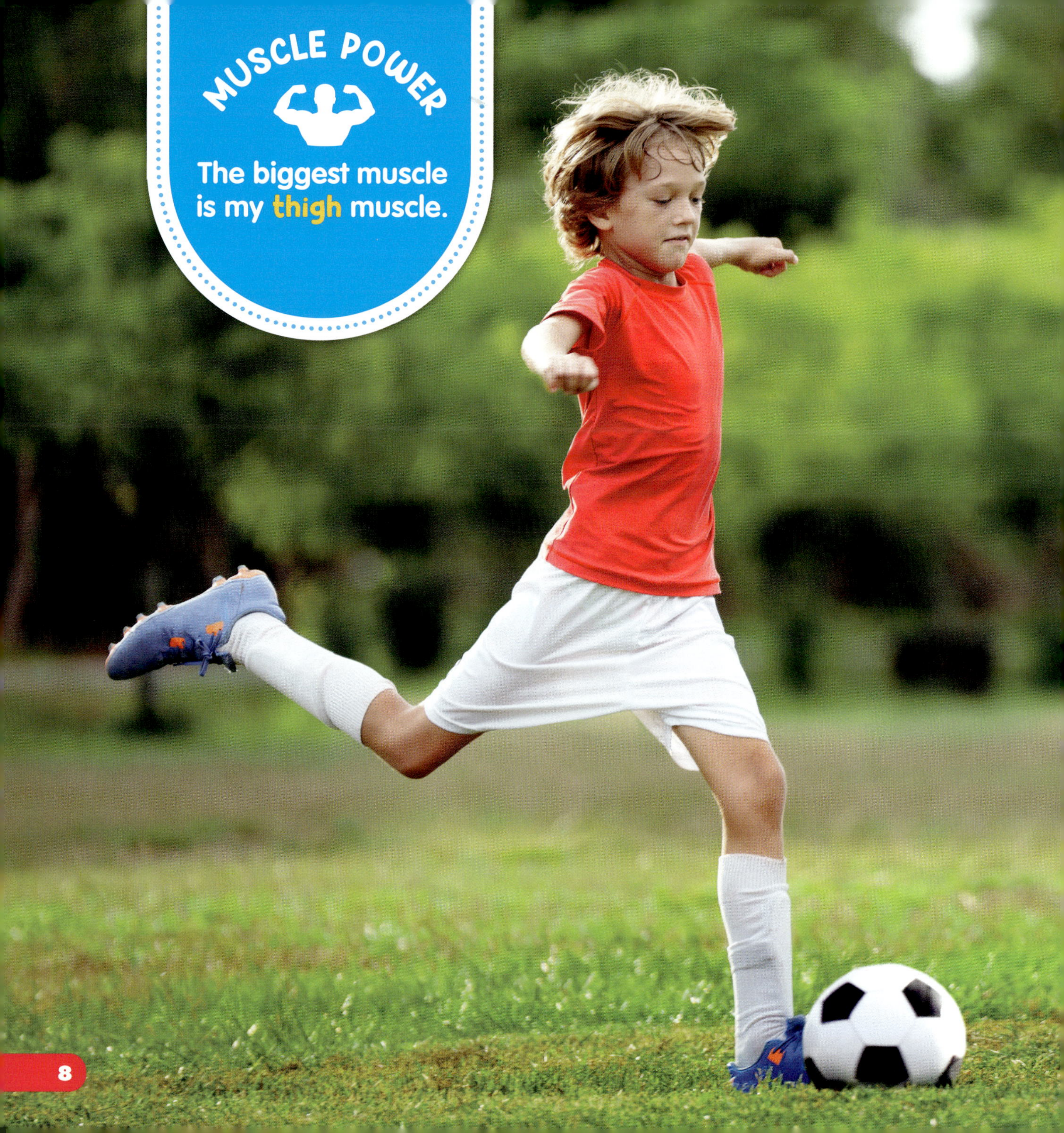

My leg muscles are big.

They help me run.

They help me jump.

They help me kick.

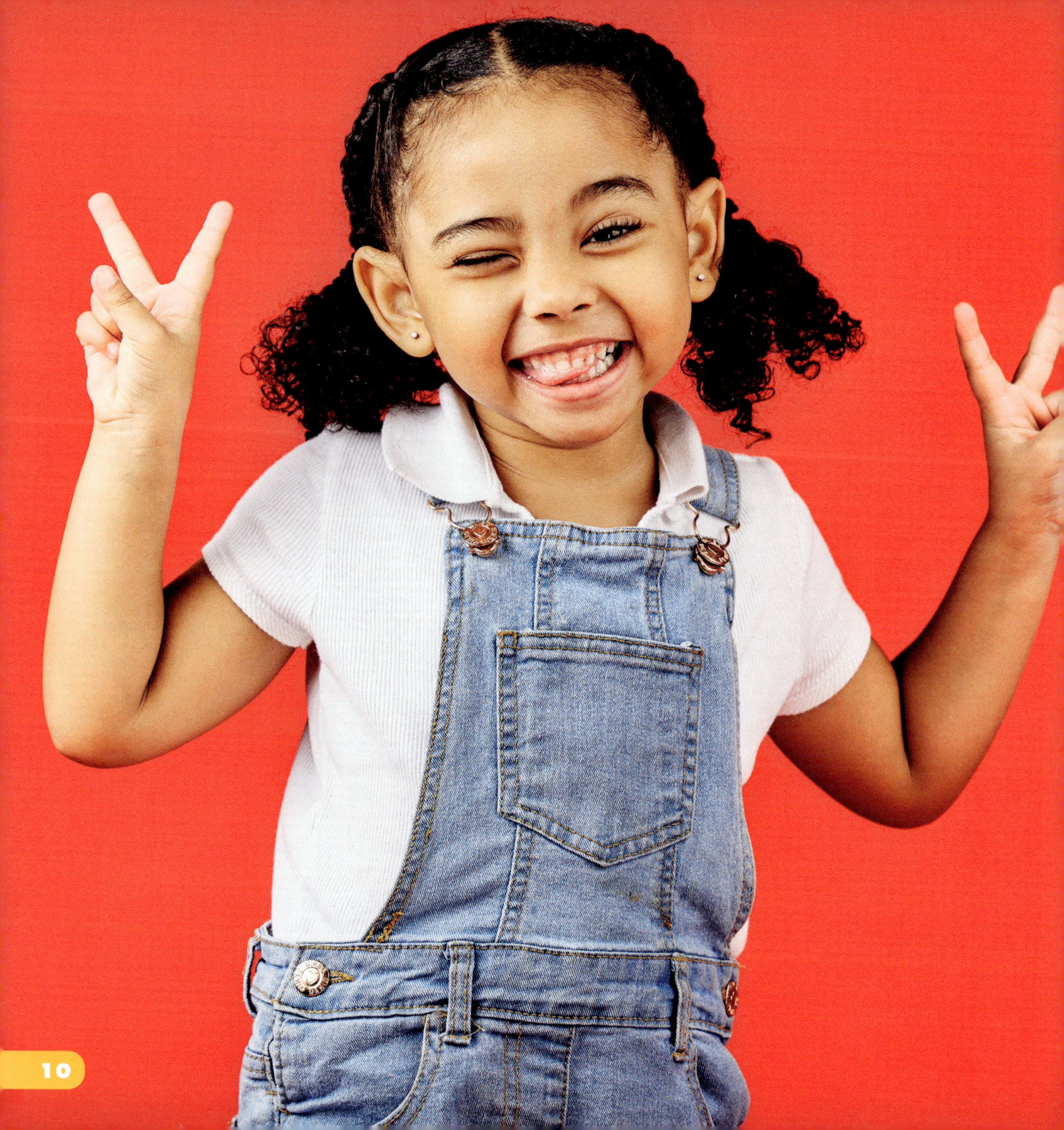

Tiny Muscles

Some muscles are small.

Tiny muscles in my eyes help me **blink**.

MUSCLE POWER

My eyelids blink about 15 times a minute.

I lift things.

I carry things.

My arm muscles help me push.

They help me pull.

They help me throw.

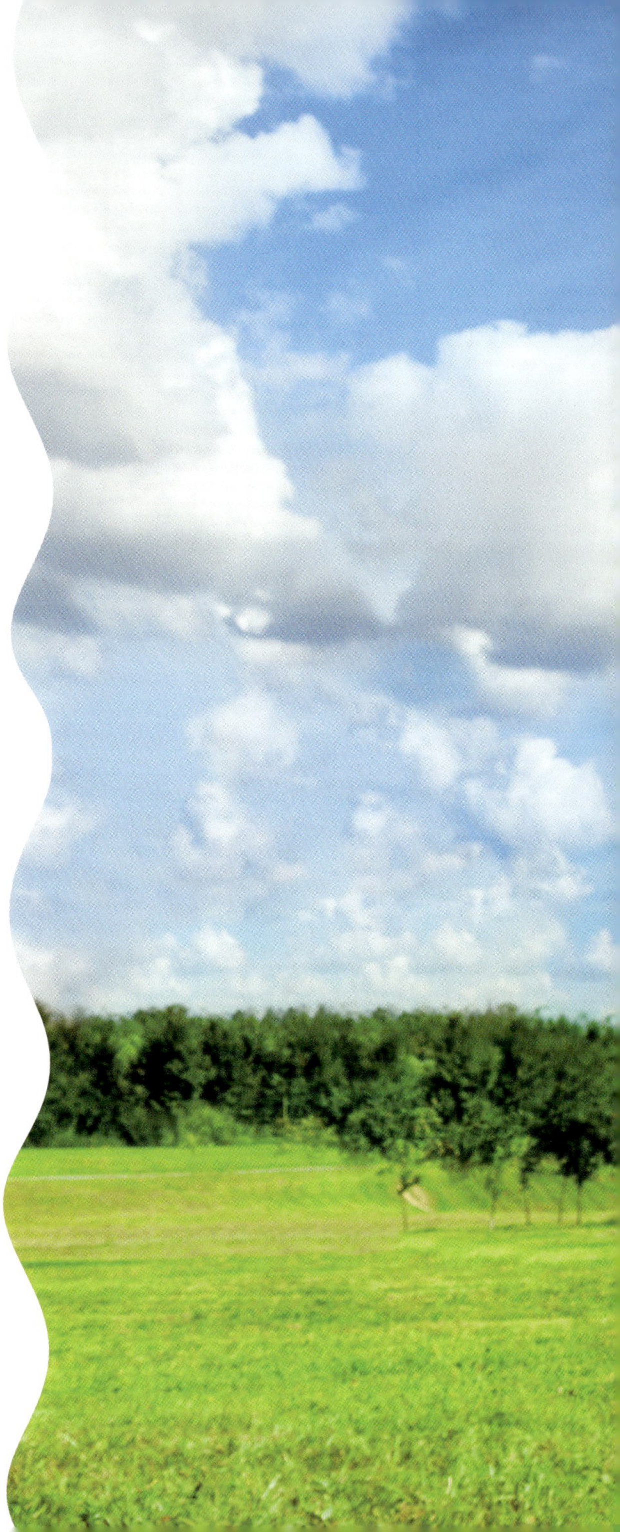

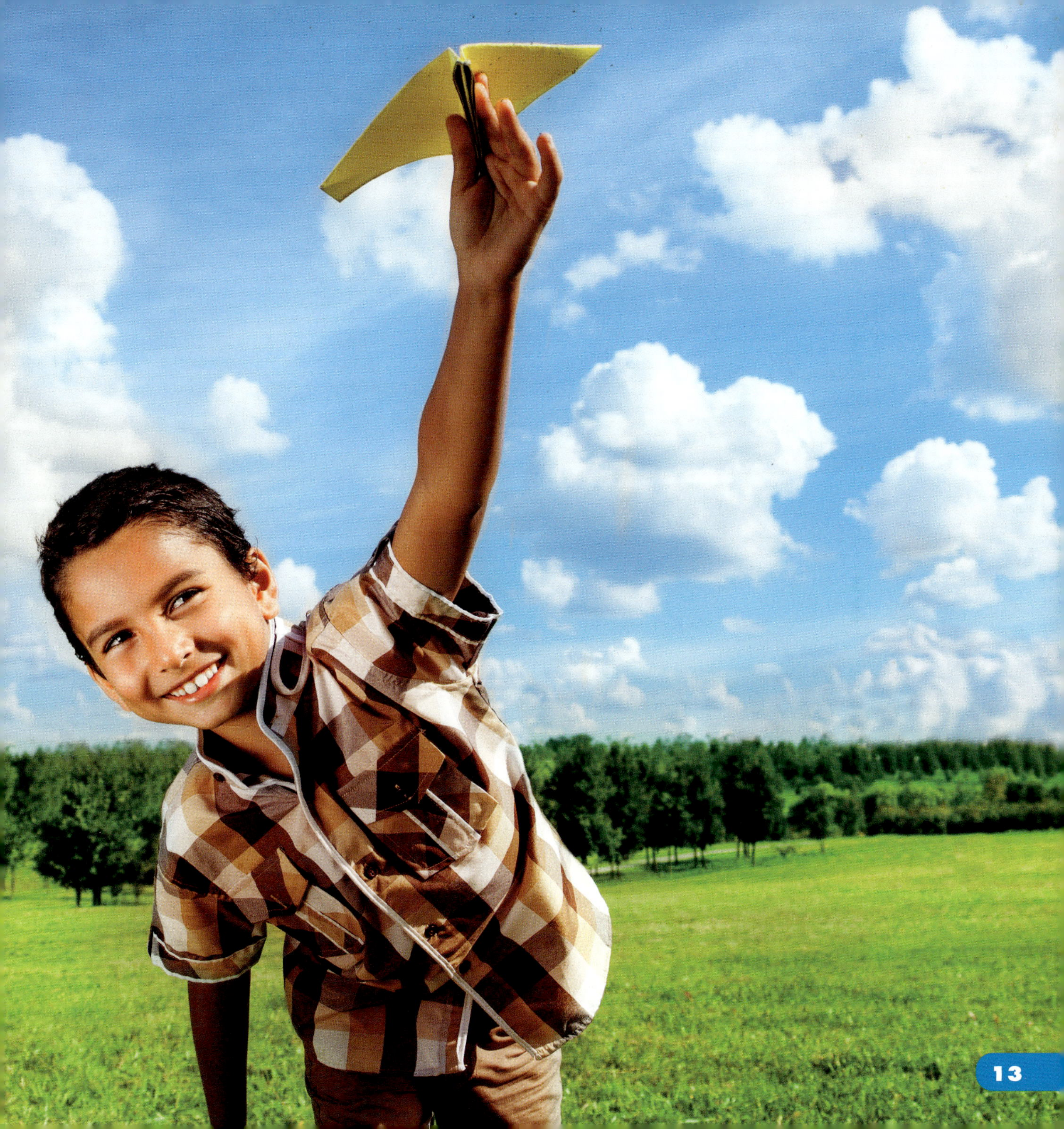

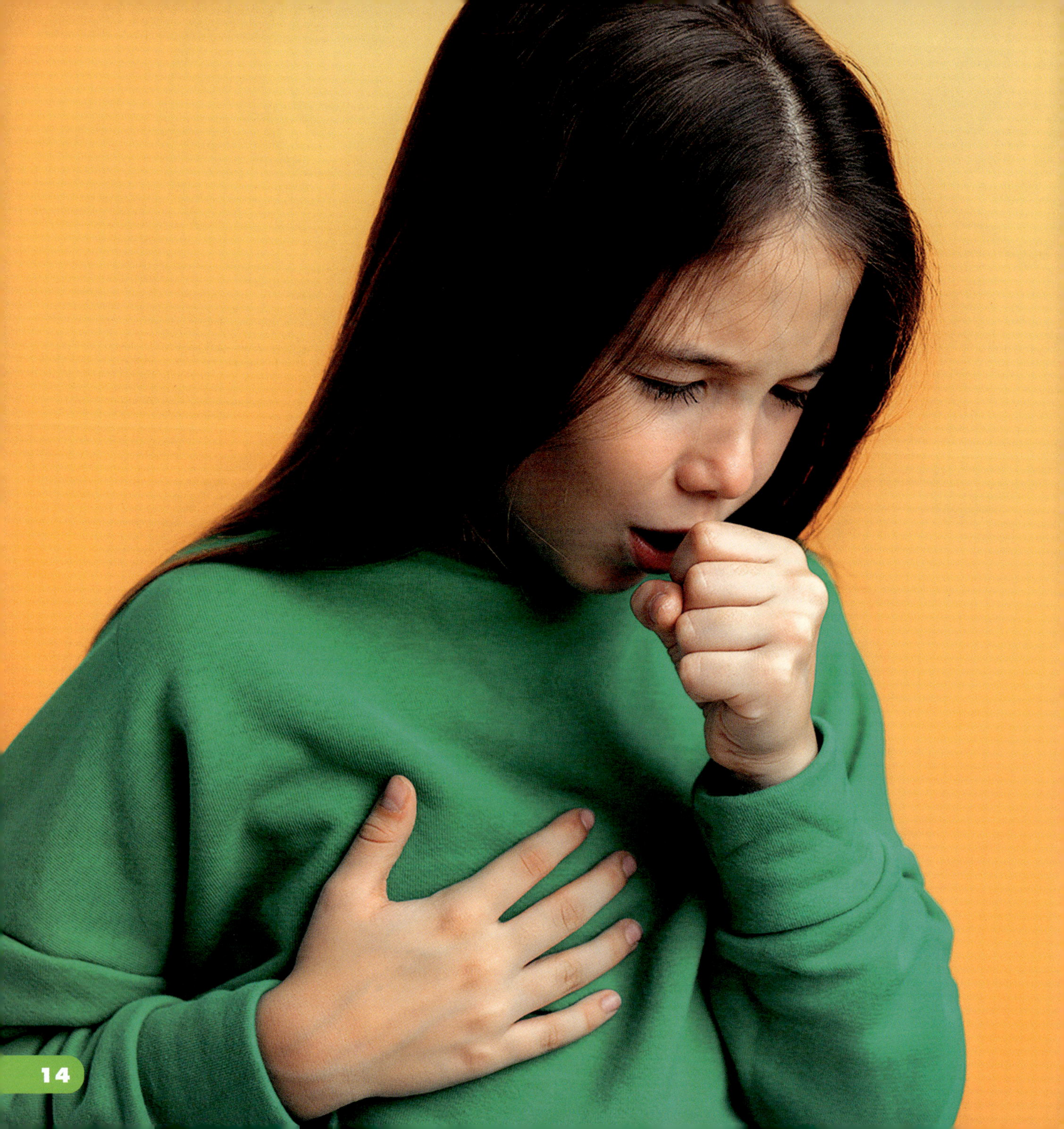

Muscles in My Tummy

My tummy muscles
help me sit up.

They help me laugh.

They help me **cough**!

MUSCLE POWER

Laughing uses 5 muscles in my tummy.

Muscles Move My Face

I **wink**. I **frown**. I smile.

Muscles in my face help me show feelings.

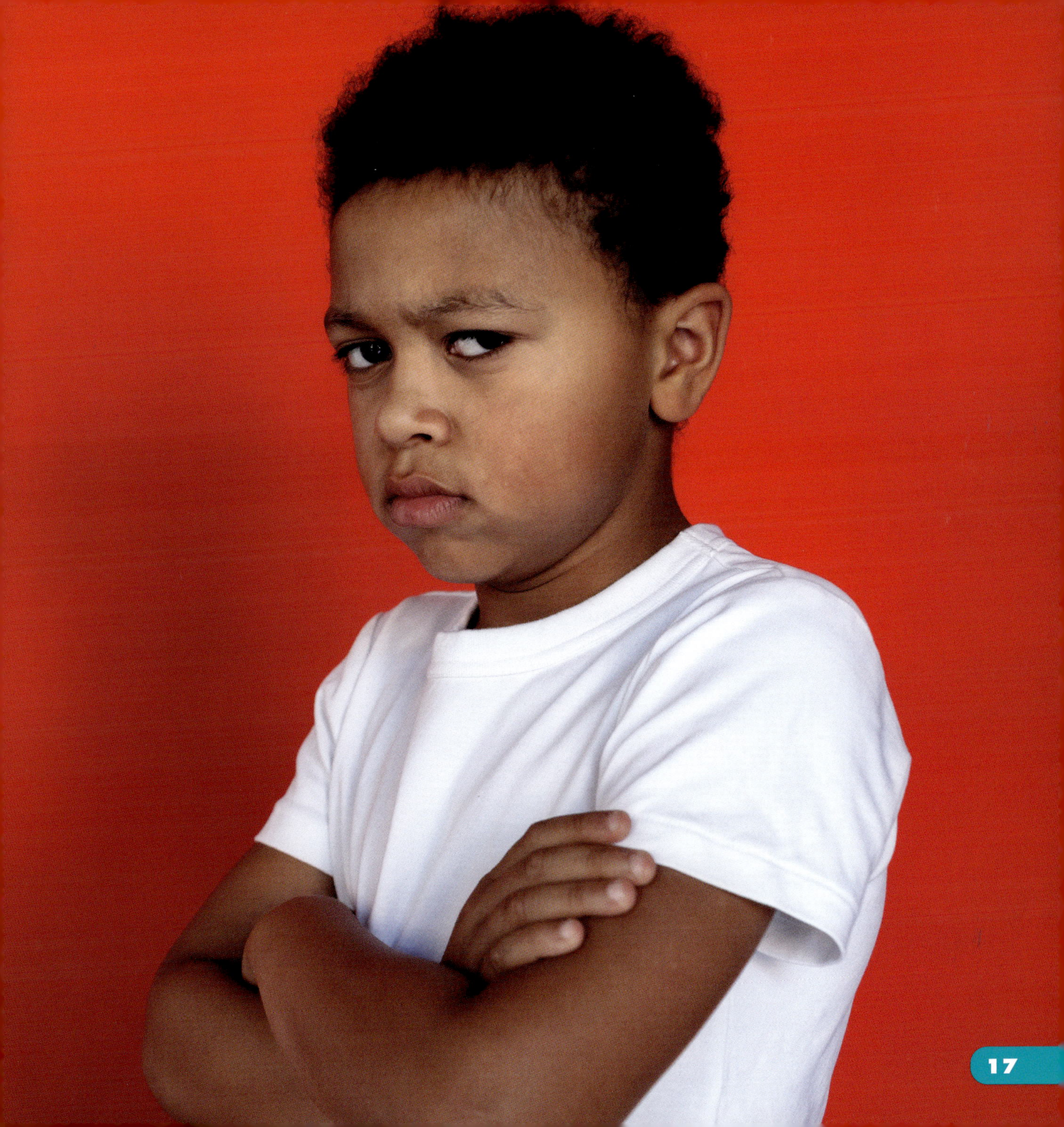

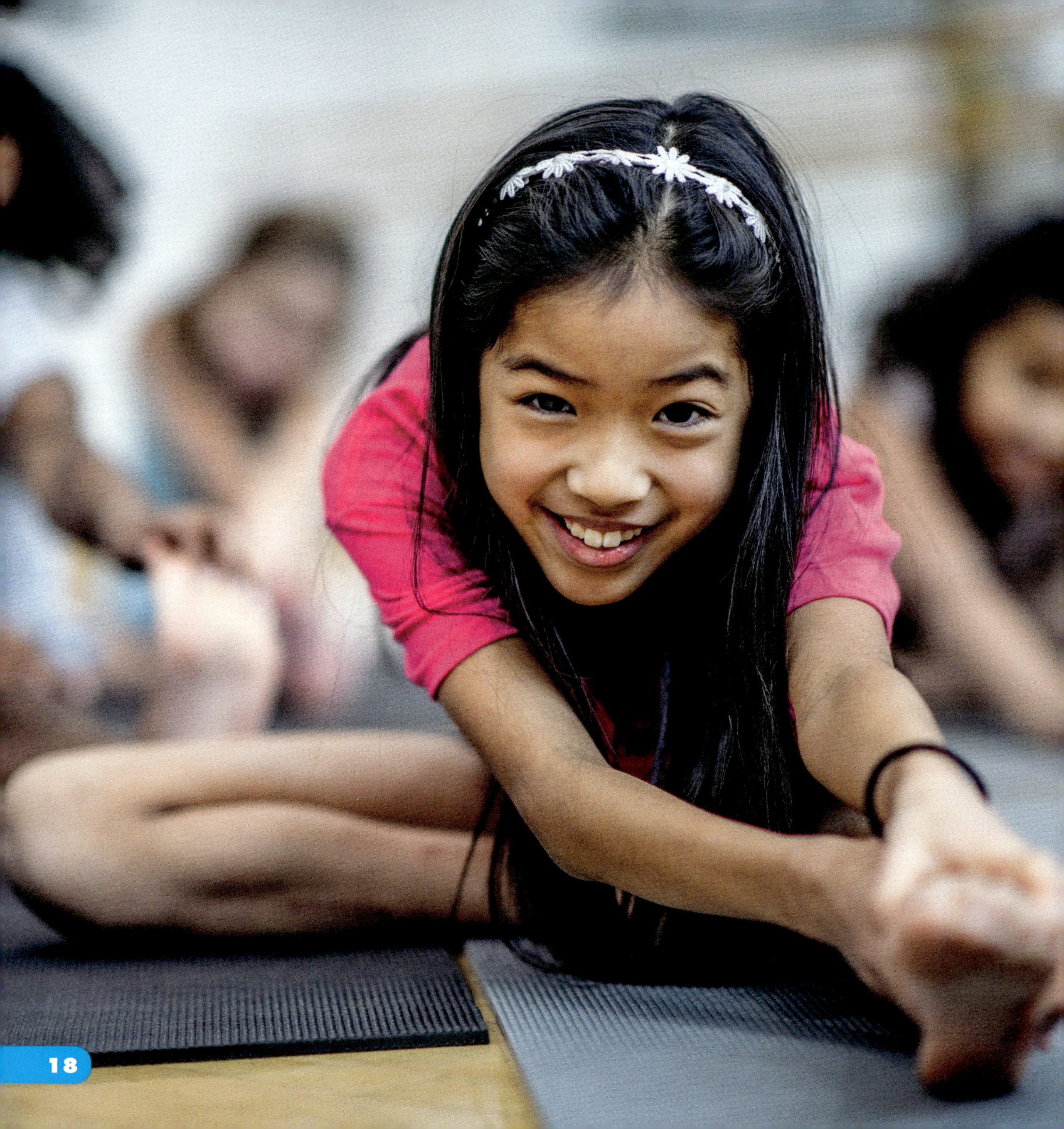

Exercise Makes Muscles Strong

I run. I jump. I stretch.

My muscles grow strong.

Exercise makes muscles happy.

Good Night Muscles

Muscles rest when I sleep.

Sleep helps my muscles grow.

Sleep keeps my muscles **healthy**.

Tomorrow, my muscles will play again!

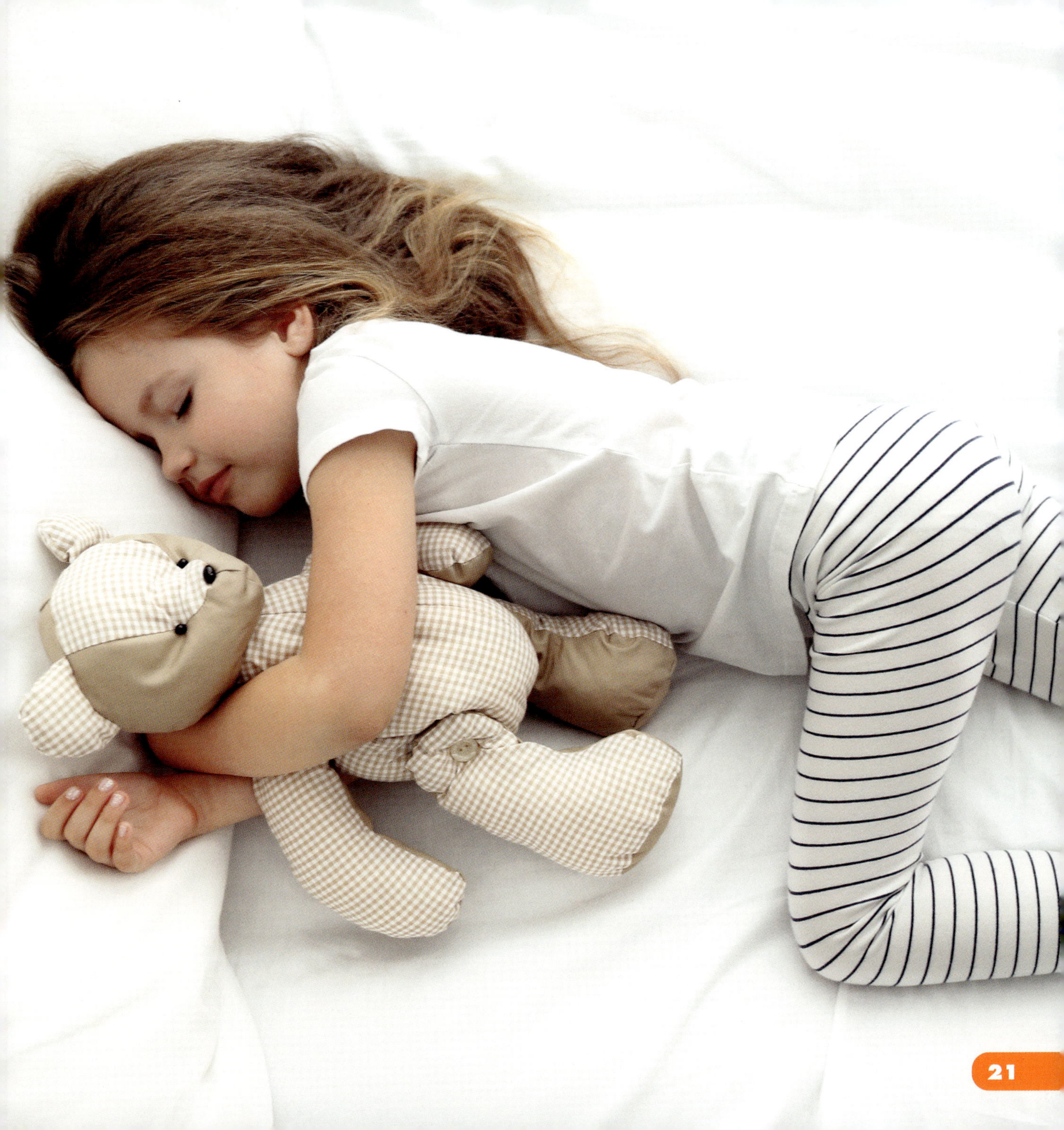

Glossary

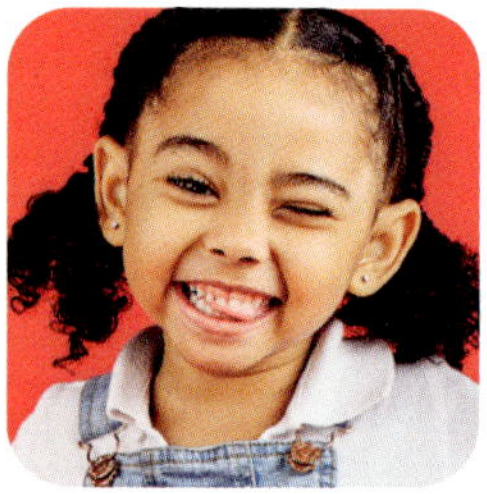

blink (blĭngk) to quickly open and close your eyes.

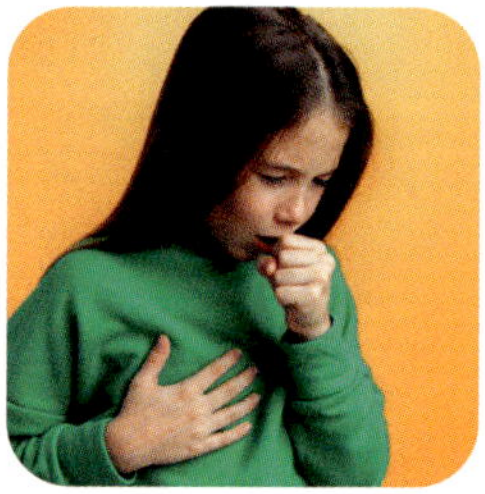

cough (kawf) A quick sound you make when your throat or chest needs to clear

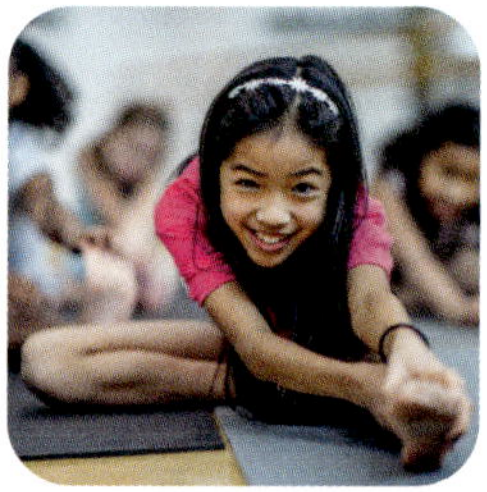

exercise (ek-ser-size) moving your body to play and stay healthy

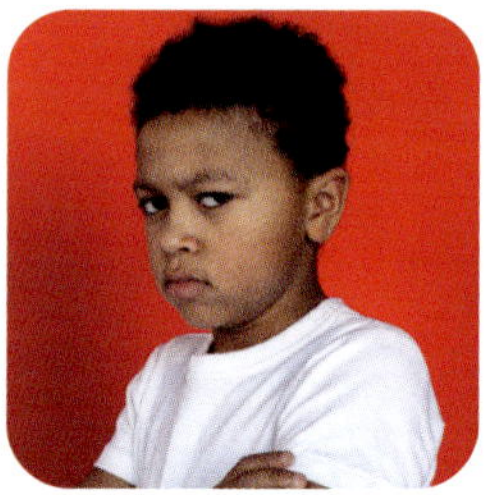

frown (fraün) to make your eyebrows go down when you are unhappy or thinking

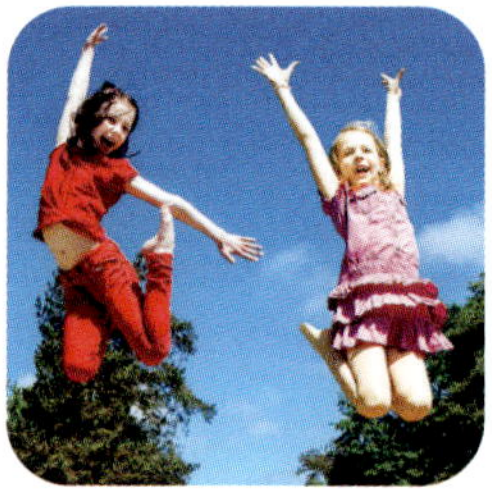

healthy (hĕl-thē) feeling good and strong in your body

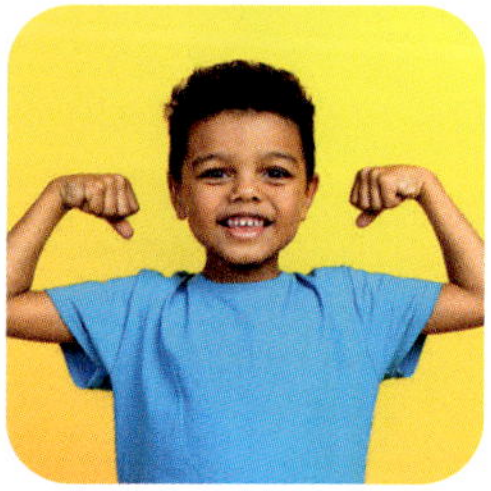

muscles (muh-sulz) parts of your body that help you move

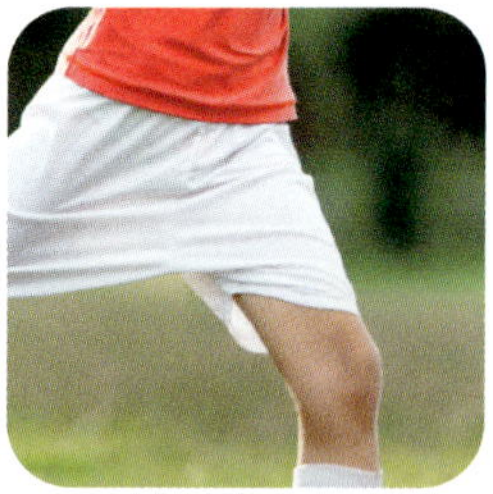

thigh (thī) the top part of your leg, between your hip and knee

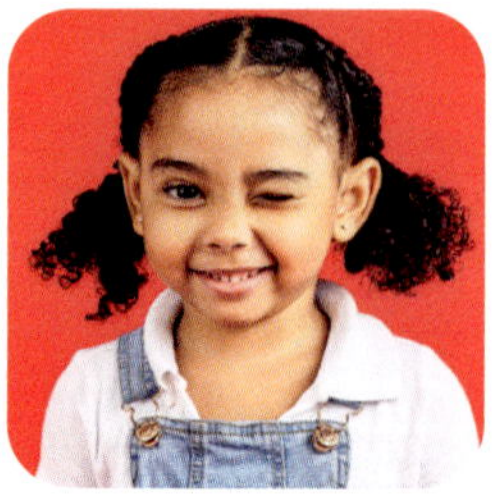

wink (wĭngk) to quickly close one eye as a signal or for fun

Quiz: My Strong Muscles

1. Muscles help me move my body.

A. Yes B. No

2. Sleep keeps my muscles healthy.

A. Yes B. No

3. Laughing uses muscles in your tummy.

A. Yes B. No

4. Exercise helps muscles get stronger.

A. Yes B. No

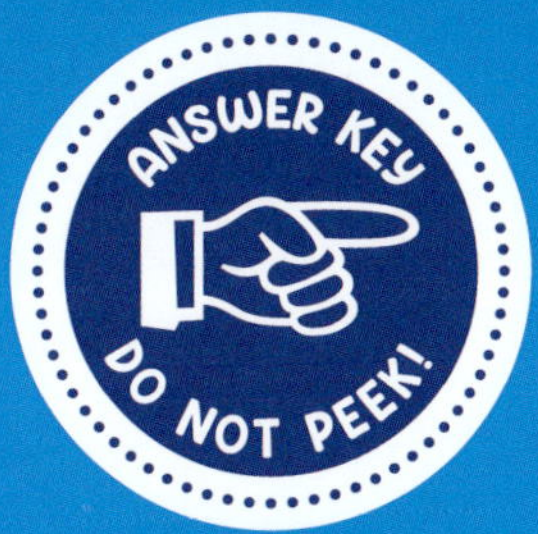

ANSWER KEY:

How many times did you answer yes?

4 Yes: Awesome! You know your muscles well.

3 Yes: Great! You learned some new facts.

2 Yes: That's okay! Keep reading.

1 Yes: You're starting to learn. Keep going!

Further Reading

Hicks, Dwayne. *Your Amazing Muscles.* Rosen Publishing, 2023

Rose, Rachel. *Muscles.* Bearport Publishing, 2022

On the Internet

Kids Discover Online—"Muscles for kid"

https://online.kidsdiscover.com/unit/muscles

A beautifully designed unit that includes fun activities and explanations of major muscles, how they work, muscle issues, and comparisons with animals.

Kids-Health—"How Does the Muscular System Work?" (Video)

https://kidshealth.org/en/kids/msmovie.html

A short, animated video that shows how muscles give us power to move, pump blood, and do jobs in our body.

Your Muscles (for Kids)—KidsHealth

https://kidshealth.org/en/kids/bones.html

A kid-friendly, age-appropriate article explaining how your muscles help you move-even when you're sitting still.

Index

About the Author

Rachel Daniels is a former elementary school teacher who loves reading and discovering new things. She lives in sunny South Florida with her husband, close to her children and grandchildren. When she's not reading or writing, she enjoys playing Canasta with friends. Her goal is to make learning exciting and joyful for young readers everywhere.